Carpal tunnel syndrome information booklet

WE ARE VERSUS ARTHRITIS

We're the 10 million people living with arthritis. We're the carers, researchers, health professionals, friends and parents all united in our ambition to ensure that one day, no one will have to live with the pain, fatigue and isolation that arthritis causes.

We understand that every day is different. We know that what works for one person may not help someone else. Our information is a collaboration of experiences, research and facts. We aim to give you everything you need to know about your condition, the treatments available and the many options you can try, so you can make the best and most informed choices for your lifestyle.

Contents

What is carpal tunnel syndrome?	4
What are the symptoms of carpal tunnel syndrome?	5
What causes carpal tunnel syndrome?	7
How is carpal tunnel syndrome diagnosed?	8
What treatments are there for carpal tunnel syndrome?	10
Self-help and daily living	15
Research and new developments	15
Where can I find out more?	16
Talk to us	17

What is carpal tunnel syndrome?

Carpal tunnel syndrome is a condition that happens when the median nerve is compressed or squeezed as it passes through the wrist (see Figure 1). This happens when the carpal tunnel inside your wrist becomes inflamed.

The median nerve controls some of the muscles that move the thumb and carries information back to the brain about sensations in your thumb and fingers.

Figure 1. The tendons and the median nerve pass through the carpal tunnel in the wrist

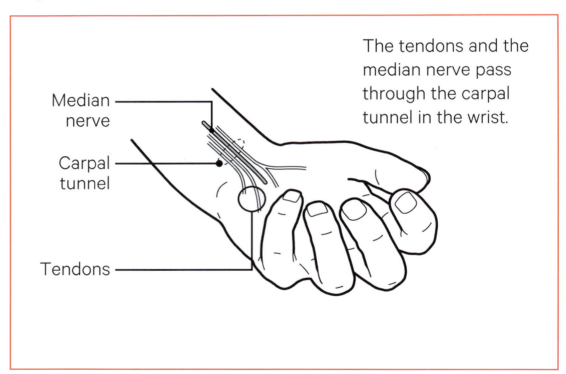

When the nerve is squeezed it can cause tingling, numbness, pain or aching in the affected hand. Women are more likely than men to develop carpal tunnel syndrome. The condition affects people of all ages, but it's more common in people over 50.

What are the symptoms of carpal tunnel syndrome?

Carpal tunnel syndrome causes a tingling feeling or pins and needles, numbness, and sometimes pain in the hand. The symptoms can sometimes be felt in the forearm or further up your arm. It tends to come on gradually over a period of weeks.

You'll usually feel it worst in the thumb, index and middle fingers, but sometimes it might feel like your whole hand is affected. You may also have an ache running up your arm to the shoulder or neck. It can affect just one or both hands.

The symptoms tend to be worse at night and can disturb your sleep, but you may also notice it when you wake up in the morning. Hanging your hand out of bed or shaking it around will often help reduce the pain and tingling.

You may not notice the problem at all during the day, though certain activities – such as writing, typing, DIY or housework – can bring on your symptoms. However, if the nerve is badly squeezed, you might have symptoms throughout the day.

Your hand might feel weak, or the fingers numb, or both. You may drop things and find that activities needing fine finger movements, such as writing or fastening buttons, become more difficult.

Figure 2. Carpal tunnel syndrome can cause numbness or tingling in the shaded area

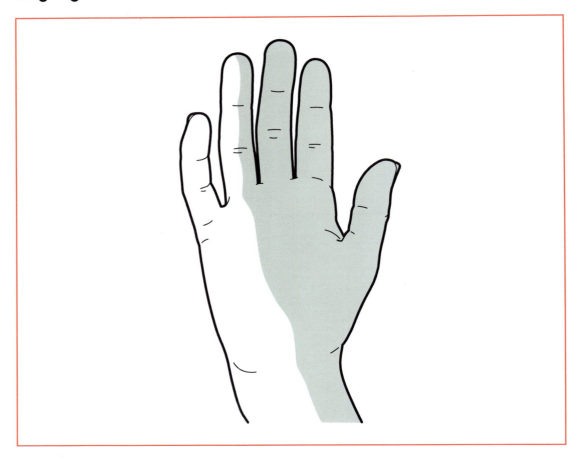

For more information on things you can do if your symptoms are causing problems with daily life, see the Versus Arthritis booklets:
Sleep and arthritis; Looking after your joints

You can view all our information online at:
www.versusarthritis.org

What causes carpal tunnel syndrome?

The median nerve is very sensitive to pressure, and it might not be possible to say what has caused the condition for you. Some of the things that can increase your risk of developing carpal tunnel syndrome are:

- any form of arthritis in the wrist, especially if there's swelling of the wrist joint or the tendons that run through the carpal tunnel
- hormonal changes, for instance during pregnancy, which can sometimes affect connective tissues and put pressure on the nerve
- the thyroid gland not producing enough hormones, sometimes called hypothyroidism or an underactive thyroid gland
- diabetes
- a wrist fracture
- your genes
- obesity
- work that places heavy demand on your wrist
- using vibrating tools
- occasionally, some medications can cause it, particularly the breast cancer treatments exemestane and anastrazole.

How is carpal tunnel syndrome diagnosed?

Examination of the wrist

Your doctor or health professional will ask you to describe your symptoms. They will take a look at your hand and wrist to assess how bad the condition is. If the wrist is swollen due to arthritis or tendon swelling, this could be the cause of your symptoms.

If you've had the condition for some time, there may be signs of muscle wasting at the base of the thumb. If the problem is severe, your thumb, index and middle fingers may be insensitive or numb to either a gentle touch or a pin prick.

Your doctor may tap over the median nerve on the palm side of your wrist – this is known as Tinel's test. Or they may ask you to bend your palm towards your forearm for up to a minute, which is known as Phalen's test. These tests can help to diagnose carpal tunnel syndrome, but they aren't reliable, so you may also have one of the tests described below.

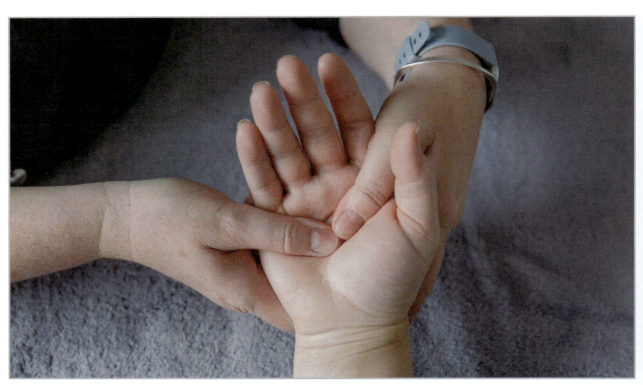

Tests

Sometimes carpal tunnel syndrome can be mistaken for something else, such as pressure on nerves in the neck due to disc problems or arthritis, which can cause similar symptoms.

A nerve conduction test may help and can be used to measure how bad the compression of the nerve is.

These tests can be done in several ways, but one common way is to see how your nerve reacts when a small electric current is put through one of your fingers. Electrodes will be attached to your skin on the fingers and wrist to measure the speed of your nerve's response to the current.

This test doesn't measure how bad your symptoms are, but it can show how badly damaged the nerve is. When the nerve is damaged, the speed at which messages travel between the finger and the wrist is slower.

Ultrasound scans are sometimes used in diagnosis, because the nerve can become swollen before it goes through the carpal tunnel and this can be seen on a scan. Ultrasounds can also show some of the causes of carpal tunnel syndrome, including swelling in the tendons or joint.

What treatments are there for carpal tunnel syndrome?

There are many different treatments for carpal tunnel syndrome, but not all of them will work for everyone.

Not all cases of the condition will cause long-term problems in the hand, and some people may find it improves without any medical treatment. If there's a particular cause for your problem, such as an underactive thyroid gland or arthritis, then your symptoms may improve by treating that.

Your doctor will talk to you about the different treatments available and help you decide which would be best for you. If the condition is severe and you're experiencing weakness in your hand muscles, then it's important to get treatment quickly, and you'll normally be advised to have surgery.

Splints

A resting splint for your wrist will often help – particularly if your symptoms are worse at night. A working splint to support your wrist that pushes the palm back slightly may be helpful if certain activities bring your symptoms on.

An occupational therapist or physiotherapist will be able to tell you about the different types of splint. Some therapists may recommend exercises of the wrist that might help prevent the median nerve becoming stuck to nearby tendons.

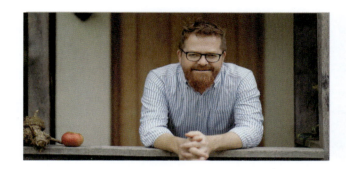

Drugs

A steroid injection will be helpful in most cases, although the effect may wear off after weeks or months. A small amount of steroid is injected into the carpal tunnel, which helps to reduce any swelling.

A steroid injection into the wrist joint itself may help if you have arthritis in your wrist. The injection might feel uncomfortable at the time, but it can be very helpful in treating carpal tunnel syndrome.

If the steroid injection is helpful but your symptoms return later, your doctor might repeat the injection. But repeated injections can become less effective or cause skin changes so they might not always be given.

Surgery

You may need surgery if there's severe compression of your median nerve or if the numbness and pain don't improve with other treatments. The surgery, known as carpal tunnel release or decompression surgery, relieves pain by reducing the pressure on your median nerve.

Surgery usually takes place as a day case, where you'll go home the same day. The operation is normally carried out under a local anaesthetic and may be done by conventional open surgery or by keyhole surgery. Your surgeon will be able to tell you which is most suitable for you.

Following the operation, you might need to wear a bandage on your hand and wrist for a few days. It's important that you keep moving your fingers and arm to reduce stiffness and swelling, and to prevent the nerve and tendons getting caught up in the scar tissue that can form after the operation. You may be able to start gentle exercises on the same day as your operation.

Your stitches will usually be taken out between 10 and 14 days after the operation, though some surgeons use dissolving stitches instead which don't need to be removed.

You should recover from the surgery in less than a month, although it may take longer to get all the feeling back in your hand, especially if you've had the condition for a long time.

Sometimes, the operation may not bring a complete recovery – especially if you have muscle wasting or loss of sensation in your hand - but it should greatly reduce your pain. If you feel there has been no improvement in your symptoms in the first six weeks after your operation, you should speak to your surgeon.

During the first few weeks after surgery you should avoid heavy tasks, but you should start to use your hand for lighter activities, as long as it's not too uncomfortable. You shouldn't drive until you are able to comfortably make a fist with your hand.

For most people this surgery is very successful. But as with all operations, there is a small risk of complications, which may include infection, nerve damage or scarring. On rare occasions, the pain may continue, or it may return some time after the operation, even if it had seemed successful at first.

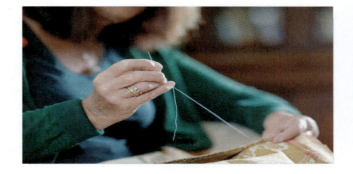

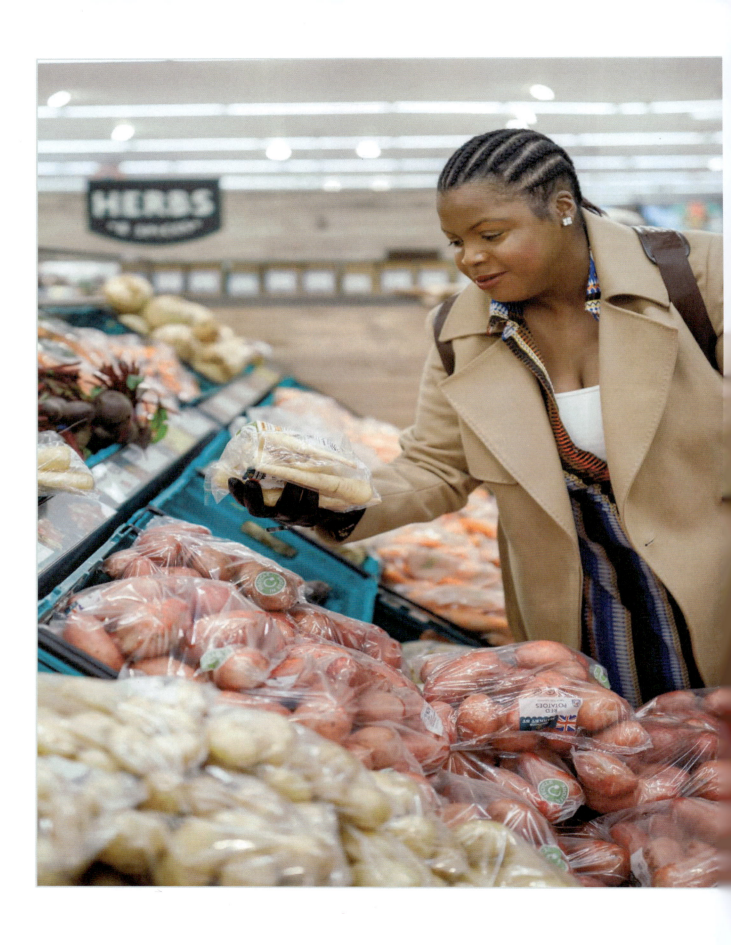

Self-help and daily living

No particular diet has been shown to help either relieve or prevent carpal tunnel syndrome. However, a healthy balanced diet and regular exercise are important for your general health.

If you think your work may be causing your symptoms you should discuss this with your supervisor or an occupational health nurse. If necessary, your local JobCentre Plus office can put you in touch with a Work Coach or Disability Employment Advisor who'll be able to tell you how changes to your equipment or working techniques could help.

For more information see the Versus Arthritis booklet:
Diet and arthritis

You can view all our information online at:
www.versusarthritis.org

For more information on Working with arthritis visit:
www.versusarthritis.org/work-and-arthritis

Research and new developments

There's ongoing research looking into treatment and managing pain for carpal tunnel syndrome. Current clinical studies are creating more effective wrist supports for people with carpal tunnel syndrome. They're also testing whether steroid injections are more helpful than night splints in reducing symptoms and improving use of the hand in the short-term.

Where can I find out more?

If you've found this information useful, you might be interested in other titles from our range. You can download all of our booklets from our website www.versusarthritis.org or order them by contacting our Helpline.

Bulk orders

For bulk orders, please contact our warehouse, APS, directly to place an order:

Phone: 0800 515 209
Email: info@versusarthritis.org

Tell us what you think

All of our information is created with you in mind. And we want to know if we are getting it right. If you have any thoughts or suggestions on how we could improve our information, we would love to hear from you.

Please send your views to **bookletfeedback@versusarthritis.org** or write to us at: **Versus Arthritis, Copeman House, St Mary's Court, St Mary's Gate, Chesterfield, Derbyshire S41 7TD.**

Thank you!

A team of people helped us create this booklet. We would like to thank Dr Ben Thompson, Dr Jeremy Bland, Dr Linda Chesterton, Sean Macklin and Marcus Bateman for helping us review this booklet.

We would also like to give a special thank you to the people who shared their opinions and thoughts on the booklet. Your contributions make sure the information we provide is relevant and suitable for everyone.

Talk to us

Helpline

You don't need to face arthritis alone. Our advisors aim to bring all of the information and advice about arthritis into one place to provide tailored support for you.

Helpline: 0800 5200 520
Email: helpline@versusarthritis.org

Our offices

We have offices in each country of the UK. Please get in touch to find out what services and support we offer in your area:

England
Tel: 0300 790 0400
Email: enquiries@versusarthritis.org

Scotland
Tel: 0141 954 7776
Email: scotland@versusarthritis.org

Northern Ireland
Tel: 028 9078 2940
Email: nireland@versusarthritis.org

Wales
Tel: 0800 756 3970
Email: cymru@versuarthritis.org

Notes

Notes

Carpal tunnel syndrome

Carpal tunnel syndrome is a condition that causes a tingling, numbness, and sometimes pain in the hand. In this booklet we explain what causes carpal tunnel syndrome and how it's treated. We also give some hints and tips on managing your carpal tunnel syndrome in daily life.

For information please visit our website:
versusarthritis.org
0300 790 0400

- /VersusArthritis
- @VersusArthritis
- @VersusArthritis

**FAMILIES
FRIENDS
DOCTORS
RESEARCHERS
SUPPORTERS
FUNDRAISERS
VOLUNTEERS
VERSUS ARTHRITIS**

Printed in Great Britain
by Amazon